HEALTHY EATING

For Extremely Busy People Who
Don't Have Time For It

Christine Hoza Farlow, D.C.

Copyright © 1997 by Christine Hoza Farlow, D.C.
All rights reserved.
Printed in the United States of America

Every effort has been made to insure the accuracy of the information presented in this book. However, nothing in this book should be construed as medical advice or used in place of medical consultation.

ISBN 0-9635635-1-3

This book is dedicated to my husband, David, and my daughter, Melissa.

ACKNOWLEDGEMENTS

I thank Dr. Barbara Van Horne and Dr. Bryan Stern for thoroughly critiquing my manuscript and offering invaluable comments that ultimately shaped this book into a form that is truly easy for the extremely busy person to use.

I thank Dr. Walter Schmitt for inspiring me with his comments and encouragement.

I thank Dr. Lendon Smith and Dr. Bruce West for taking time from their busy schedules to review my unsolicited manuscript and return their comments promptly.

I thank Michael Van Meter of Royal Publications, for discussing this book with me when it was barely an idea, and for his continued support and encouragement.

I especially thank my husband, David, for his love and support from beginning to end, for his numerous edits and re-edits of my manuscript, and for his patience and tact in our numerous discussions of this book.

I thank my little daughter, Melissa, for letting Mommy work when she would rather have my attention.

Last but not least, I thank everyone else who supported me and encouraged me in the long process of conceiving this book in my mind to the completion of it in its final form.

CONTENTS PAGE

The "KISS" for Health Books................................	1

SECTION I	Quick Start To Healthy Eating	3

What Is Healthy Eating?...	5
Recommendations For Healthy Eating.....................	7
What To Eat, What To Avoid.............................	7
Your Personal Food Planner...................................	20
The 43-Second Rule...	22
Why Most People Fail To Eat Healthfully And	
How You Can Avoid It...................................	22
How To Put Together Quick Meals...................	22
Sample Quick Meals...	26
Developing Good Eating Habits That Last A	
Lifetime...	33

SECTION II	More Quick Facts About Healthy Eating	37

Nutrients...	39
Protein...	39
Carbohydrates..	44
Fat...	47
Vitamins and Minerals....................................	49
Fiber...	53
Water..	53
The Healthy Eating For Extremely Busy People Food	
Pyramid..	56
Adulterated Food: Food Additives, Pesticides and	
Irradiation..	62
Food Additives...	62
Pesticides...	66
Irradiation..	67
How To Read Labels...	69
Eating Out...	81
Food Combining...	83
References...	85

The "KISS" For Health Books

The purpose of the "Keep It Simple Series For Health" books is to provide you with brief, practical and simple information on a variety of health and nutrition topics.

These books are for you if you are

- a health conscious individual who doesn't have the time or the desire to read in depth on the subject

- just beginning to explore health and nutrition and don't quite know where or how to start

The books are designed to be brief, but with enough detail so you can stay healthy with hardly any effort at all.

This is the first in a series of books designed to give you easily usable information to improve your health and well being. Other books are currently in progress. Call, fax or e-mail for more information. See the back of the book for the phone numbers and e-mail address.

SECTION I

QUICK START TO HEALTHY EATING	PAGE
What Is Healthy Eating	5
Recommendations For Healthy Eating	7
What To Eat, What To Avoid	7
Your Personal Food Planner	20
The 43 Second Rule	22
Why Most People Fail To Eat Healthfully And How You Can Avoid It	22
How To Put Together Quick Meals	22
Sample Quick Meals	26
Developing Good Eating Habits That Last A Lifetime	33

WHAT IS HEALTHY EATING

Health is not just the absence of disease. It is a state of well being in body, mind and spirit. If you are truly healthy, you will feel vibrantly alive, full of energy and have a zest for life.

You are unique. There is no one way of eating that is right for everyone. But there are certain foods that are generally healthy and certain foods that are generally unhealthy. This book will help you find what is healthy for you.

Eating nourishes your body and gives it the proper fuel so you can function optimally.

When you drive a car, you put gasoline in the gas tank. If you put water or soda in the gas tank, your car wouldn't run. Your body needs the same kind of attention you give your car. It needs the proper fuel to run efficiently.

If you don't take care of your car and it breaks down beyond repair, you can buy a new car. If you don't take care of your body and it breaks down and gets sick or diseased, you can't get a new body.

However, the good news is that, up to a point, your body is very forgiving. If you abuse your body and it gets sick or diseased, it will give you a second, a third or even more chances to care for it properly. And with the proper care, your body can return to a state of health. But you never know when you've used up all your chances. So why take the risk!

To truly attain a state of real health, you have to feed your body the right kind of fuel. **Here are the three keys to healthy eating:**

1. Eat the right kinds of foods to
    - supply your body with healthy proteins, carbohydrates and fats

- get the vitamins and minerals your body needs

2. Eliminate or minimize the use of foods
    - that have been sprayed with pesticides
    - that contain food additives
    - that have been highly processed
    - that have been irradiated or have irradiated ingredients

3. Drink plenty of "good" water.

And remember my "80-20 Rule." If you're good 80% of the time, you can give yourself an occasional "treat."

If you're under the care of a doctor, check with your doctor first before you decide to use the "80-20 Rule." You may have to "be good" 100% of the time for a period of time until you're healthy enough to enjoy a "treat."

So, get your car in gear and let's travel to our first stop on the road to *healthy eating* – **What To Eat and What To Avoid.** ⇨⇨⇨

RECOMMENDATIONS FOR HEALTHY EATING

What To Eat	What To Avoid
Fruit	
<ul><li>fresh</li><li>dried without<ul><li>sulfur</li><li>preservatives</li><li>additives</li><li>sweeteners</li></ul></li><li>frozen without<ul><li>preservatives</li><li>additives</li><li>sweeteners</li></ul></li><li>canned in it's own juice (infrequently)</li></ul>	<ul><li>*canned in*<ul><li>*light syrup*</li><li>*heavy syrup*</li></ul></li><li>*dried with*<ul><li>*sulfur dioxide*</li><li>*sweeteners*</li><li>*preservatives*</li></ul></li><li>*frozen with*<ul><li>*preservatives*</li><li>*sweeteners*</li></ul></li></ul>
Vegetables	
<ul><li>fresh<ul><li>raw</li><li>lightly steamed</li><li>baked</li><li>broiled</li></ul></li><li>frozen without<ul><li>preservatives</li><li>other additives</li></ul></li></ul>	<ul><li>*canned*</li><li>*frozen with*<ul><li>*preservatives*</li><li>*other additives*</li></ul></li><li>*fried*</li><li>*overcooked*</li></ul>

What To Eat	What To Avoid

- sprouts
  - alfalfa
  - lentil
  - mung
  - sunflower	

Grains	

- all whole grain products should be free of
  - sugar
  - chemical additives
  - preservatives
- whole grains
  - amaranth
  - barley
  - brown basmati rice
  - brown rice
  - buckwheat
  - bulgur
  - millet
  - oats and oatmeal
  - quinoa
  - rye
  - wheat
  - wild rice
- whole grain products
  - bread
  - muffins
  - tortillas
	- *all grain products with*
	  - *white flour*
	  - *unbleached flour*
	  - *enriched flour*
	  - *sweeteners*
	  - *chemical additives*
	- *refined and processed grains*
	  - *white rice*
	  - *quick oats*
	  - *instant oatmeal*
	  - *instant cereals*
	- *refined and processed grain products*
	  - *white bread*
	  - *wheat bread (if it's not "whole" wheat)*
	  - *soft breads*
	  - *muffins*
	  - *crackers*
	  - *cookies*
	  - *pastries*

What To Eat	What To Avoid
<ul><li>cereals (unsweetened)</li><li>pasta</li><li>crackers</li><li>sprouted grain products<ul><li>bread</li><li>muffins</li><li>tortillas</li></ul></li><li>corn tortillas made with<ul><li>corn only</li><li>corn, lime and water</li></ul></li></ul>	<ul><li>*baked goods*</li><li>*breakfast cereals*</li><li>*pasta made from*<ul><li>*white flour*</li><li>*semolina flour*</li><li>*enriched flour,*</li><li>*other processed grains*</li></ul></li></ul>

Legumes

<ul><li>dry<ul><li>beans</li><li>peas</li><li>lentils</li><li>chickpeas</li></ul></li><li>canned legumes prepared without<ul><li>animal products</li><li>chemical additives</li></ul></li><li>soy products<ul><li>tofu</li><li>tempeh</li><li>miso</li><li>soy milk</li></ul></li></ul>	<ul><li>*canned beans prepared with*<ul><li>*animal fat*</li><li>*sweetener*</li><li>*chemical additives*</li></ul></li><li>*pork and beans*</li></ul>

What To Eat	What To Avoid
<td colspan="2" align="center">Nuts and Seeds (refrigerate)</td>	

- raw nuts
  - almonds
  - filberts
  - pine nuts
  - cashews (sparingly)
- raw seeds
  - sunflower seeds
  - pumpkin seeds
  - sesame seeds
- raw nut butters
  - almond
  - sunflower
  - cashew (sparingly)
  - sesame or tahini
	- *roasted*
	  - *nuts*
	  - *seeds*
	- *dry roasted*
	  - *nuts*
	  - *seeds*
	- *peanuts*
	- *peanut butter*

<td colspan="2" align="center">Soups</td>	

- home made with
  - fresh vegetables
  - grains
  - legumes
- canned (infrequently) without
  - sweetener
  - chemical additives
	- *canned with*
	  - *MSG*
	  - *Sweetener*
	  - *chemical additives*
	- *dried with*
	  - *MSG*
	  - *sweetener*
	  - *chemical additives*
	- *bouillon cubes*

What To Eat	What To Avoid
Eggs	

- from chickens that are
  - hormone free,
  - antibiotic free
  - fed all natural feed
 	
- refrigerated
 	
- prepared by
  - poaching
  - soft boiling
  - hard boiling
	- *from chickens that have been fed*
	  - *hormones*
	  - *antibiotics*
	
	- *unrefrigerated*
	
	- *raw*
	
	- *prepared by*
	  - *frying*
	  - *pickling*

Meat and Poultry	

- 1 - 4 ounce servings
 	
- from animals that are
  - organically grain fed
  - chemical free
  - antibiotic free
 	
- poultry
  - chicken
  - turkey
 	
- once a week or less
  - lean lamb
  - lean beef
	- *more than 4 ounces at a meal*
	
	- *animals fed*
	  - *hormones*
	  - *antibiotics*
	
	- *pork*
	
	- *processed meats*
	  - *luncheon meats*
	  - *hot dog,*
	  - *sausages*
	  - *bacon*
	  - *smoked meats*

What To Eat	What To Avoid
• wild game	• pickled meats • organ meats
Fish	

• deep ocean fish
  • salmon
  • sardines
  • mackerel
  • sea trout
  • red snapper
  • halibut
  • ocean perch
  • sole
  • albacore tuna
  • cod
  • flounder
  • swordfish
  • haddock
  • whiting
• tuna
  • packed in water
  • no broth
  • no chemical additives
	• fresh-water fish
	  • rainbow trout
	  • lake trout
	  • catfish
	  • smelt
	  • mullet
	  • carp
	  • pike
	  • bass
	  • lake perch
	  • bream
	• canned in oil or broth
	• shell fish
	• raw fish
	• salted fish
	• fried fish
	• herring
	• anchovies

What To Eat	What To Avoid
Fats and Oils	
<ul><li>extra virgin olive oil</li><li>raw organic flax seed oil</li><li>cold pressed or expeller pressed oils<ul><li>canola oil</li><li>sesame oil</li><li>sunflower oil</li></ul></li><li>butter--mix 50-50 with canola oil for "better butter"</li></ul>	<ul><li>*hydrogenated and partially hydrogenated oils*<ul><li>*hardened oils*</li><li>*margarine*</li></ul></li><li>*cottonseed oil*</li><li>*refined processed oils*</li><li>*saturated fats*<ul><li>*shortening,*</li><li>*lard*</li><li>*coconut oil*</li><li>*palm kernel oil*</li></ul></li></ul>
Beverages	
<ul><li>pure water<ul><li>filtered</li><li>reverse osmosis</li></ul></li><li>tea<ul><li>herbal, caffeine free</li><li>green tea</li></ul></li><li>juices<ul><li>fresh vegetable</li><li>fresh fruit - dilute 50-50 with good pure water</li><li>bottled organic juices</li></ul></li></ul>	<ul><li>*tap water*</li><li>*alcohol*</li><li>*caffeinated beverages*<ul><li>*coffee*</li><li>*tea*</li><li>*some herbal teas*</li></ul></li><li>*carbonated beverages*<ul><li>*soda*</li><li>*diet drinks*</li></ul></li></ul>

What To Eat	What To Avoid
<ul><li>no sweeteners</li><li>no additives</li><li>frozen organic juices</li><li>no sweeteners</li><li>no additives</li></ul>	<ul><li>*fruit drinks (not 100% juice)*</li><li>*juices, sweetened*</li><li>*breakfast drinks*</li></ul>
Dairy Products	
<ul><li>soy yogurt</li><li>non-dairy beverages<ul><li>rice</li><li>oat</li><li>soy</li><li>almond</li></ul></li></ul>	<ul><li>*all cow's milk products*<ul><li>*milk*</li><li>*buttermilk*</li><li>*cheese*</li><li>*cottage cheese*</li><li>*sour cream*</li><li>*ice cream*</li><li>*yogurt*</li><li>*kefir*</li></ul></li></ul>
Sweeteners	
<ul><li>unsweetened organic fruit juice (non organic is concentrated with the pesticides used on the fruit)</li><li>unsweetened applesauce</li><li>rice amasake</li><li>sucanat (dehydrated cane-juice crystals)</li><li>date sugar</li></ul>	<ul><li>*sugar*</li><li>*brown sugar*</li><li>*powdered sugar*</li><li>*corn syrup*</li><li>*high fructose corn syrup*</li><li>*raw sugar*</li><li>*turbinado sugar*</li></ul>

What to Eat	What To Avoid

• rice-syrup powder
• brown rice syrup
• barley malt
• sorghum syrup
• stevia
• aguamiel
• organic fruit juice concentrate (non organic is concentrated with the pesticides used on the fruit)
• pure maple syrup
• blackstrap molasses
• fructose
• pure raw honey (not for children under 18 months of age)
• fructooligosaccharides (FOS)
• all sweeteners are best used sparingly or avoided
	• *beet sugar*
	• *buttered syrup*
	• *caramel*
	• *carob syrup*
	• *dextrose, sucrose*
	• *honey (cooked or processed)*
	• *molasses (except blackstrap molasses)*
	• *all artificial sweeteners, including:*
	  • *aspartame*
	  • *Equal*
	  • *Nutrasweet*
	  • *Sweet 'n Low*
	  • *Saccharin*
	  • *Acesulfame potassium*
	  • *Sunette*
	  • *Mannitol*
	  • *Sorbitol*
	  • *Xylitol*
	  • *Sorbitol*
	  • *Xylitol*
	  • *Hydrogenated starch hydrosylate*

What To Eat	What To Avoid
\multicolumn{2}{c}{Seasonings}	

What To Eat	What To Avoid
Seasonings	
<ul><li>Celtic sea salt</li><li>Herbamare</li><li>seaweed seasonings<ul><li>dulse</li><li>kelp</li></ul></li><li>herbs and spices (non-irradiated)</li><li>cayenne pepper</li><li>soy sauce, tamari</li><li>Dr. Bragg's Liquid Aminos</li></ul>	<ul><li>*common table salt*</li><li>*black pepper*</li><li>*white pepper*</li><li>*MSG*</li><li>*irradiated herbs and spices*</li></ul>
Condiments	
<ul><li>ketchup substitute<ul><li>sugar free</li><li>chemical free</li></ul></li><li>mustard<ul><li>sugar free</li><li>chemical free</li></ul></li><li>mayonnaise<ul><li>no sugar</li></ul></li></ul>	<ul><li>*ketchup with*<ul><li>*added sugar*</li><li>*chemical additives*</li></ul></li><li>*mustard with added*<ul><li>*sugar*</li><li>*chemical additives*</li></ul></li><li>*mayonnaise with*<ul><li>*sugar*</li></ul></li></ul>

What To Eat	What To Avoid

• no hydrogenated or partially hydrogenated oils
• no chemical additives
 	
• jams and jellies
  • fruit juice sweetened
  • no chemical additives
	• *hydrogenated or partially hydrogenated oils*
	• *chemical additives*
	
	• *jams and jellies with*
	  • *added sugar*
	  • *chemical additives*
	
	• *sauces with*
	  • *sweeteners*
	  • *MSG*
	  • *other chemical additives*
	
	• *other condiments with*
	  • *sweeteners*
	  • *chemical additives*

Snacks and Convenience Foods	

• potato chips (infrequently)
  • baked
  • no chemical additives
 	
• fake french fries - bake instead of frying
 	
• carob, unsweetened
 	
• baked goods
  • fruit juice sweetened
  • whole grain flours
	• *potato chips*
	
	• *french fries*
	
	• *sweets*
	  • *chocolate*
	  • *candies*
	
	• *baked goods*
	  • *sweetened*
	  • *refined flours*
	  • *chemical additives*

What to Eat	What to Avoid
• no chemical additives	• *gelatin desserts* • *fad foods* • *fake foods* • *diet foods* • *frozen dinners*

- **Eat organically grown food** when possible. A Rutgers University study titled "Variations in Mineral Content in Vegetables" concluded that "Commercially grown inorganic vegetables are very low in mineral and trace mineral content." The study compared non-organic vegetables purchased from the supermarket with organic vegetables grown in naturally fertilized soil. Organic food is also free of chemicals and pesticides.

- **Read labels.** Buy foods where the ingredients are "food" ingredients, not chemical additives.

- If there's anything you like to eat that's not included in **What To Eat** or **What To Avoid**, read the label. If it has any ingredients that are not common food items, it's probably not good for you. If you need help reading the ingredients on the label, get *FOOD ADDITIVES: A Shopper's Guide To What's Safe & What's Not (see page 86).*

The next stop is **Your Personal Food Planner**. Use this effectively and you'll assure your success in eating healthfully. Let's go. ⇨⇨⇨

YOUR PERSONAL FOOD PLANNER

Your Personal Food Planner is designed to help you develop healthy eating habits that last a lifetime. It will help keep you focused on eating healthy foods you like – healthy foods that are acceptable substitutes for the unhealthy foods you like.

The key to your success in developing healthy eating habits is to substitute **healthy foods you like** for the unhealthy foods you like.

Copy the Personal Food Planner form so you can use it over and over again.

Here's how to use Your Personal Food Planner:

1. Choose one or two foods
   - you like to eat that are unhealthy **and**
   - you are ready and willing to eliminate

   Write them in the **Foods I like to eat that I should avoid** column.

   If you're not ready to eliminate certain unhealthy foods you like to eat, find some you are ready to eliminate. This will make it a lot easier for you to be successful in your healthy eating adventure.

2. Next, choose some healthy foods to substitute for the unhealthy foods you are ready to eliminate. Choose foods that
   - you already know you like and/or
   - you would like to try

   Write them in the **Healthy foods I can substitute** column.

3. Keep doing this until you have eliminated all the unhealthy foods you like to eat, and eating healthfully has become so automatic you don't have to think about it any more.

PERSONAL FOOD PLANNER

Foods I like to eat that I should avoid	Healthy foods I can substitute

THE 43-SECOND RULE

Why Most People Fail To Eat Healthfully And How You Can Avoid It

This rule states you have 43 seconds to find something healthy to eat after you've noticed you're hungry. If you can't find something healthy to eat, you'll eat just about anything.

This means that you must have meals or snacks that are already prepared or that you can quickly and easily prepare. If you don't, you probably won't be eating healthy most of the time. However, this is not as difficult as it sounds. Here's...

How To Put Together Quick Meals

The key to being able to put together meals quickly is to have
- certain key food items on hand all the time
- the kitchen tools to help with speedy preparation

Here is a sample list of some foods and kitchen items. You can add to it or subtract from it based upon the healthy foods you like to eat and the food preparation tools you like to use.

Fruit
- fresh fruit
- frozen fruit (without added sweetener or food additives)
- raisins
- avocados
- lemons
- limes

Breads
- whole grain bread
- sprouted grain flourless bread
- corn tortillas (corn only, or corn, water and lime)
- whole wheat tortillas (no additives or preservatives)

- sprouted wheat tortillas
- rice cakes

Salad vegetables
- leaf lettuce
- salad mix (combination of leaf lettuces and salad greens prewashed in a package—not iceberg lettuce)
- tomato
- cucumber
- celery
- radishes
- jicama
- carrots
- zucchini
- onions
- bell pepper (green, red, yellow)
- sprouts

Cooking vegetables
- broccoli
- string beans
- summer squash
- frozen peas (no additives or preservatives)
- frozen corn (no additives or preservatives)
- garlic
- potatoes
- sweet potatoes

Grains
- brown rice
- millet
- quinoa

Cereals
- oatmeal
- puffed rice cereal (brown rice only - no other ingredients)

- puffed millet cereal (millet only - no other ingredients)
- puffed corn cereal (corn only - no other ingredients)

Pasta
- whole grain pasta
- natural pasta sauce (no sugar, preservatives or other chemical additives)

Legumes
- split peas
- lentils
- dried beans
- canned beans (pinto, pink, black, kidney, garbanzos, etc., cooked in water with no chemical additives)
- tofu

Oils
- extra virgin olive oil
- flaxseed oil
- sesame oil (cold pressed)
- canola oil (cold pressed)
- sunflower oil (cold pressed)

Nuts and Seeds - raw
- sunflower seeds
- pumpkin seeds
- sesame seeds
- almonds
- filberts
- cashews (sparingly)
- pine nuts
- most nuts except peanuts

Nut Butters
- almond
- cashew (use sparingly)

- sunflower
- sesame butter or tahini

Meat and Fish
- whole fryer (hormone-free, antibiotic-free)
- tuna (canned in water—no other ingredients)

Condiments
- raw unfiltered apple cider vinegar
- salsa (no sugar, chemical additives)
- tamari
- Braggs Liquid Aminos
- mayonnaise (no sugar, hydrogenated or partially hydrogenated oils, chemical additives)
- mustard (no sugar, chemical additives)

Beverages
- rice milk
- soy milk
- oat milk
- green tea
- herbal teas (caffeine free)
- unsweetened 100% fruit juice
- pure water

Kitchen Utensils
- good sharp knives
- cutting board
- vegetable steamer (stainless steel)
- food processor (must at least shred and chop)
- blender
- stainless steel or glass cookware
- pressure cooker (nice, but not essential)

SAMPLE QUICK MEALS

Breakfasts

- ❖ Rice Cakes & Fruit
  - fresh or frozen fruit, eaten first
  - rice cakes with nut butter and raisins

- ❖ Protein Smoothie
  - rice, oat or soy milk,
  - banana,
  - fresh or frozen berries or peaches,
  - 2 tbsp. protein powder
  - blend in a blender

- ❖ Bagel & Fruit
  - fruit or fruit juice,
  - sprouted whole grain bagel with butter or nut butter

- ❖ Cereal & fruit
  - fruit or fruit juice
  - puffed millet cereal with rice milk

- ❖ Soy Yogurt & Muffin
  - plain soy yogurt with fresh fruit,
  - whole grain muffin,

Add your own healthy favorites that you discover here

Lunches

- ❖ Veggie Salad Taco
    - corn tortillas thinly spread with sesame tahini or almond or cashew butter
    - add some beans or tofu
    - top with left over salad with flax or olive oil and raw unfiltered apple cider vinegar dressing

- ❖ Chicken and Salad Taco
    - corn tortilla thinly spread with natural mayonnaise and/or mustard,
    - add some left over chunks or slices of roasted chicken (hormone and antibiotic free)
    - top with left over salad with flax or olive oil and fresh lemon or lime juice dressing

- ❖ Avocado Sandwich and Raw Veggies
    - whole grain or sprouted grain bread
    - spread with natural mayonnaise and/or mustard
    - add avocado slices
    - then add onions, cucumber, tomato and alfalfa sprouts
    - celery and carrot sticks on the side

- ❖ Tofu Sandwich with Raw Veggies
    - whole grain or sprouted grain bread
    - spread with natural mayonnaise and/or mustard
    - add tofu slices, plain or sautéed in tamari
    - then add onions, cucumber, tomato and lettuce
    - raw cut up veggies on the side

❖ Tuna Salad and Vegetable Strips
   - drain tuna, mix with fresh lemon juice or a little natural mayonnaise, chopped celery and onion, parsley flakes
   - put on a rice cake or wrap in a corn tortilla with lettuce and tomato
   - raw carrot and zucchini strips

Add your own healthy favorites that you discover here

Dinners

- ❖ Oil-less Stir Fry, Millet and Cucumber Salad
  - Stir Fry
    - 1 cup millet, 2 cups of water, simmer until the tiny grains pop open and all water is absorbed
    - place a small amount of water in a large skillet or electric fry pan and add cut up potatoes (with the skin) and carrots
    - add sliced cabbage and onions, broccoli florets and tofu or black beans (beans, water and salt, no chemical additives) after the potatoes and carrots are just starting to get a little soft on the outside
    - simmer until broccoli is tender, but still crisp
    - serve the vegetables over the millet
  - Cucumber Salad
    - slice a cucumber, add a few slices of onion
    - dress with extra virgin olive oil or flax oil (optional), raw unfiltered apple cider vinegar and Celtic sea salt

- ❖ Rice, Beans & Veggies with Tossed Salad
  - brown rice, cooked
  - can of organic white or pinto beans, warmed
  - steamed carrots and cauliflower
  - combine and season with Celtic sea salt or Herbamare
  - tossed salad
    - prewashed salad mix (not iceberg lettuce)
    - other salad vegetables of your choice
    - toss with olive oil or flax oil and raw unfiltered apple cider vinegar, season with Celtic sea salt and dulse or herbs of your choice

- ❖ Fish Dinner & Cabbage Salad
  - baked fish with lemon juice (in a baking dish, sprinkle fish with lemon juice, cover with foil, bake at 350° until flaky)
  - baked potato
  - steamed broccoli
  - shredded cabbage and carrots with olive oil and lemon juice dressing, season with Celtic sea salt or Herbamare

- ❖ Pasta & Salad
  - whole grain pasta
  - marinara sauce (no sugar, chemical additives),
  - steamed green beans,
  - tossed salad or cucumber salad

- ❖ Fake Pizza & Cucumber Salad
  - Fake mini pizzas
    - rice cakes or toasted whole grain bread
    - topped with crumbled tofu
    - organic spaghetti or marinara sauce, or salsa (no sugar or chemical additives)
    - sliced olives, onions, green pepper, or toppings of your choice
    - sprinkled with Italian herbs (non-irradiated)
    - broil 5-10 minutes
  - Cucumber Salad – cucumber, tomato and onion tossed with flax seed oil, raw unfiltered apple cider vinegar, Celtic sea salt and dulse

Add your own healthy favorites that you discover here

Snacks

- ❖ Trail Mix
  - raw sunflower seeds and/or almonds mixed with raisins

- ❖ Rice Cakes with
  - nut butter
  - salsa
  - better butter
  - plain

- ❖ Fruit

- ❖ Avocado Dip with Cut Up Raw Veggies
  - 1 ripe avocado, mashed
  - 1-3 tsp. onion, finely chopped
  - raw unfiltered apple cider vinegar or lemon juice to taste
  - Celtic sea salt or Herbamare
  - mix and dip your choice of veggies

Add your own healthy favorites that you discover here

Add more of your own healthy favorites that you discover here.

Now, let's go find out how to make *healthy eating* a lifetime habit and see how that's going to help assure your success even more.
⇨⇨⇨

DEVELOPING GOOD EATING HABITS THAT LAST A LIFETIME

Making The Transition: Making It Work For You

Healthy eating is not just good for you. There are definite benefits you will experience when you make a habit of healthy eating, and make it a lifetime habit. You will
- feel better
- look better
- stay younger looking
- have more energy
- think more clearly
- have a stronger immune system
- reduce the risk of cancer, heart disease and other diseases
- live longer and be healthy to enjoy it

There are two ways of changing your eating habits:
- gradually
- cold turkey

In general, gradually is the easier and more permanent way of doing it.

Go to **Your Personal Food Planner** on page 20.
- Make a list of the foods that you know are unhealthy for you that you like to eat.
- Then make a list of healthy foods that you like or would like to try that you can substitute for the unhealthy foods.
- Then every day or every other day, choose one or more unhealthy foods to eliminate and substitute one or more of the foods from your *healthy foods* list.
- Keep doing this until you have eliminated all the unhealthy foods that you eat.

Do this at a pace that is comfortable for you. If you go too fast, you may be eating healthier food faster, but you may also feel deprived or like you are on a diet, and then revert back to your old eating habits after a period of time. So find your pace, be steady and consistent, and you'll be successful at developing healthy eating habits.

And remember my "80-20 rule."
- If you're good 80% of the time, you can treat yourself every once in awhile.
- Please note: If you are under a doctor's care, please check with your doctor first before you follow the "80-20 rule."

If you totally blow it,
- take a deep breath
- go back to **Your Personal Food Planner** and look at the lists you made
- start all over again with the gradual method, substituting the foods that sound the most appealing and the easiest to start making a habit of eating

Always pat yourself on the back for each positive step you make in the direction of healthier eating habits. **You don't have to do it perfectly, you just have to start doing it, and do it consistently.**

Healthy eating can take on different forms. There are a number of different philosophies about healthful eating. There is no one way or philosophy of healthy eating that will work for every individual. Everyone is unique, and different things work for different people.

Healthy eating should be looked at as a habit, not a diet. Diets don't work. You don't stay on diets for a lifetime. A diet is a temporary phenomenon. A habit is something you develop gradually over a period of time. Habits last a long time. Habits are hard to break. So you want to develop healthy eating habits.

Developing healthy eating habits should be looked at as an adventure. You're exploring new foods and new ways of eating. When you go exploring, generally you meet and examine one or a few new things in a single exploration. Rarely are you dropped into a 100% new adventure with nothing familiar to relate to.

So your healthy eating habit adventure will most likely be most successful if you
- transition into it gradually rather than jumping into it "cold turkey"
- have fun doing it!

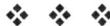

This is the end of your "Quick Start" adventure and the beginning of a new adventure in healthy eating. **Take a few minutes each day to add to your "Personal Food Planner." Keep this book handy and refer to it often.**

If you want to know more, continue on to the **More Quick Facts About Healthy Eating** adventure. Read it all the way through, or use it as a reference. Let's go. ⇨ ⇨ ⇨

SECTION II

MORE QUICK FACTS ABOUT HEALTHY EATING   PAGE

Nutrients   39
- Protein   39
- Carbohydrates   44
- Fats   47
- Vitamins and Minerals   49
- Fiber   53
- Water   53

The Healthy Eating For Extremely Busy People Food Pyramid   56

Adulterated Food: Food Additives, Pesticides And Irradiation   62
- Food Additives   62
- Pesticides   66
- Irradiation   67

How To Read Labels   69

Eating Out   81

Food Combining   83

References   85

NUTRIENTS

Protein

Protein serves many important functions in your body. Here's some basic facts about protein:
- It supplies your body with the building blocks for all your body tissues.
- It helps to form new tissues in the body, as well as to maintain and repair injured cells and tissues.
- It helps produce hormones which control metabolism, growth and development and other bodily functions.
- It helps maintain the acid-alkaline balance in the blood and the tissues - if your body is unable to maintain the proper acid-alkaline balance, you become sick.
- It helps regulate the water balance of the body - consumption of too much protein can cause dehydration.
- It is an energy source if you're not getting enough fats and carbohydrates.
- More is required in times of physical, mental or emotional stress.
- More is required for pregnant and lactating women.

If you consume 30 to 40 grams of protein a day, you should get enough protein to supply your body's protein needs, and you should avoid the dangers associated with excess protein consumption.

Children's daily protein needs vary according to age:
- 1-3 years - 23 grams
- 4-6 years - 30 grams
- 7-10 years - 34 grams
- 11-14 years - 45 grams

You can more than adequately supply your body's protein needs by eating a variety of plant foods. However, some people do very well on a vegetarian diet and some people seem to want or need animal protein. There is some research that indicates that blood type may be related to an individual's ability to be a healthy vegetarian or an individual's need for animal protein to feel healthy.

- Type A and A/B's make good vegetarians, but it's important to transition gradually from a meat-eating diet.
- Type O's may feel a need for animal proteins like eggs or fish on a daily basis.
- Type B's may want to alternate between eating vegetarian meals and animal protein meals.

However, researchers agree that Americans, in general, whether meat eaters or vegetarians, get more protein than necessary.

Too Much Protein

Too much protein is dangerous and
- is stored as fat
- can cause kidney damage because the kidneys are overworked in eliminating protein by-products
- can cause dehydration, calcium deficiency, kidney stones, osteoporosis
- can be a factor in gout, cancer, heart disease, obesity and liver disease

If you eat animal protein - meat, fish, dairy or eggs - two or three times a day, you're probably getting too much protein. The chart below gives the amount of protein per gram and per 4 ounce serving of the different animal proteins.

	Grams of protein per ounce	grams of protein in a 4 ounce serving
Red meat	6-7	24-28
Poultry	3-4.5	12-18
Fish	5-8	20-32
Milk	1	4
Cheese	3-12	12-48

One large egg provides 6 grams of protein.

It doesn't take a lot of figuring to see that one meal containing animal protein can provide a whole day's worth of protein or more.

Too Little Protein

Symptoms of protein deficiency are :
- irritability
- loss of endurance
- weight loss
- low immune response
- anemia
- poor healing
- muscle weakness
- fatigue
- retarded growth
- sugar cravings

If you feel fatigued or have low energy and endurance when you consume 30-40 grams of protein per day, **and** if eating more protein makes you feel better, then you probably need more protein.

If you crave sugar when you eat 30-40 grams of protein per day, it could mean that you need more protein, especially if you don't crave sugar when you eat more protein.

If eating more protein doesn't help, you may
- not be digesting your food
- be deficient in the B vitamins
- have a blood sugar problem

In this case you should consult with a holistic, nutritionally - oriented doctor.

Sources of protein

Protein can be animal or vegetable.

Vegetable protein can be obtained by eating a variety of plant foods: legumes, grains, nuts or seeds, fresh vegetables, and fruits.

There is no need to combine the different plant foods to make "complete proteins" at each meal.

Soybean products are a very good source of high quality vegetable protein. The utilization of soy protein in the body is comparable to the utilization of meat and poultry. Here are some soybean products:
- Tofu is a complete protein and is highly utilized by the body.
- Tempeh is a fermented soy protein product and is even higher in protein than tofu.
- Miso is a soy protein that contains digestive enzymes and live lactobacillus. This makes it very easily digestible.

The chart below lists some vegetable proteins with the amount of protein in a cup:

Vegetable protein	Grams of protein per cup	Vegetable protein	Grams of protein per cup
Tempeh	31	Black-eyed peas *	13
Soybeans *	29	Soy milk (plain)	10
Lentils *	18	Quinoa *	11
Black beans *	15	Peas *	8
Chickpeas *	15	Bulgur *	6
Kidney beans *	15	Broccoli *	5
Lima beans *	15	Brown rice *	5
Pinto beans *	14	Spinach *	5

* Cooked
(Modified from *Prescription for Dietary Wellness* by Phyllis Balch, C.N.C. used with permission)

Animal proteins include:
- eggs
- poultry
- dairy products
- meat
- fish

Egg is the protein most efficiently utilized by the human body. It is 95% utilized, compared with meat and poultry, which are only 67% utilized. Contrary to popular belief, eating eggs is not a major cause of elevated cholesterol, and avoiding eggs will not lower your cholesterol. In fact, eggs contain the nutrients which help your body to utilize cholesterol.

Eating animal protein can be harmful. Here are some of the harmful effects animal proteins can have on your body:
- Animal feed commonly contains hormones and antibiotics. When you eat
  - meat
  - eggs
  - poultry
  - dairy products

  you consume the hormones and antibiotics from the animal feed, which may
  - increase cancer risk
  - cause children to enter puberty early
  - render your body resistant to antibiotics
- Meats are very high in phosphorus. This can cause
  - a calcium-phosphorus imbalance in the body
  - the body to take calcium from the bones to maintain the calcium-phosphorus balance in the blood
  - the bones to weaken
- Eating meat is now considered a major contributing factor in
  - cancer
  - heart disease
  - other major degenerative diseases
- When children eat a lot of animal protein regularly, there is evidence that degenerative changes that occur in cancer and heart disease start occurring in children's bodies. Reducing animal proteins and adding more vegetable proteins to children's diets can prevent this.
- Eating dairy products can cause
  - allergies
  - asthma
  - canker sores
  - insulin-dependent diabetes
  - respiratory problems
  - skin problems
- Fish are contaminated with industrial waste, toxic metals and agricultural runoff.

- Eating contaminated fish may increase cancer risk.
- Fish from the open ocean tend to be less contaminated than fresh-water fish
- Farm grown fish may be contaminated with drugs, vaccines, hormones and pesticides. Eating these fish may also increase cancer risk
- Pan frying and charcoal broiling can cause the formation of carcinogens, or cancer-causing agents, in meat.

Here are some healthier ways of eating animal products:
- Meat, poultry, eggs, or dairy products
    - choose the products that come from organically grain fed, drug-free and chemical-free animals
    - eat red meat not more than once a week
    - eat small portions, one to four ounces at a meal
    - eat wild game, it is lower in fat and is drug and chemical free
    - remove the fat from red meat
    - remove the skin from poultry
- Fish
    - eat no more than 4 ounces at a meal once or twice a week
    - choose fish from the open ocean, they are less contaminated than fresh-water fish (*see page 12*)
    - buy frozen fish to reduce the chances of bacterial contamination
- Eat meat, fish or poultry not more than once a day.
- Eggs can be eaten 3 or more times a week, even daily if they are from hormone free and drug free chickens
- Dairy products should be eaten rarely or not at all.
- **Safe methods for cooking**
    - meat are roasting, stewing, steaming or poaching
    - eggs are poaching, boiling
    - fish are baking, broiling or poaching; season with raw garlic or fresh lemon juice before cooking to lower the risk of your body absorbing toxins from the fish

Carbohydrates

Carbohydrates are the body's chief source of energy. There are two kinds of carbohydrates:
- simple carbohydrates
- complex carbohydrates

Simple carbohydrates are also called the simple sugars.

They include **all** sugars, including, but not limited to:
- white sugar
- honey
- molasses
- milk sugar
- brown sugar
- fructose
- barley malt
- xylitol
- corn syrup
- maple syrup
- turbinado sugar
- sorbitol.

Simple carbohydrates also include:
- white rice
- refined flour products
- white corn grits

Refined flour is
- white flour
- bleached flour
- wheat flour.
- enriched flour,
- unbleached flour

If it does not say "whole" wheat flour, it is refined and low in vitamins and minerals, and fiber. Refined flour is used in breads, bagels, pasta, pastries, and other baked goods.

Simple carbohydrate foods:
- give a quick burst of energy followed by a quick drop in energy
- cause you to want to eat more and more of the simple carbohydrate food
- are generally low in nutritional value
- contain little in the way of vitamins, minerals and fiber

It is best to avoid the simple carbohydrates.

Exception: Fruits and fruit juices are
- simple carbohydrates that are good for you
- rich in vitamins and minerals
- high in nutritional value

Fruit sugars are metabolized more slowly than refined sugars.

Here are some guidelines for consuming fruits and fruit juices.
- Eat fresh whole fruit. It contains valuable fiber, which is essential for a healthy bowel and lowers the risk of cancer and heart disease.
- Drink fresh fruit juices. They retain more vitamins and minerals from the fresh fruit than canned or bottled juices.
- Frozen juices are generally heat treated, which alters the taste and reduces the nutritional value.
- Canned and bottled juices are generally pasteurized, which alters the taste and reduces the nutritional value.
- Unsweetened fruit juice is preferable to
    - sweetened fruit juice
    - fruit drinks
    - sodas
    - carbonated beverages
- Dilute all fruit juices 50-50 with water to reduce the natural sugars in the juice. Remember that one 8 ounce glass of fruit juice is made from approximately 4-6 pieces of the whole fruit with none of the fiber.

Complex carbohydrates are starches, which include
- whole grains
- legumes
- vegetables

Whole grains include, but are not limited to,

• whole wheat	• brown rice	• oats
• amaranth	• quinoa	• millet
• buckwheat	• bulgur	• barley
• rye	• wild rice	

Whole grains can be found in cereals, breads and pastas. Whole grains can be cooked, combined with vegetables and eaten as a main course, or a side dish in any meal.

Legumes include
- beans
- tofu
- tempeh
- peas
- soy milk
- miso
- lentils
- chickpeas

Legumes are both starch and protein. Legumes can be cooked and eaten as part of a meal, or can be used in soups, casseroles and stews.

Vegetables:
- All vegetables, especially tubers, like potatoes, onions, turnips, rutabagas, carrots, and green leafy vegetables are high in complex carbohydrates.
- Eat mostly fresh vegetables and avoid canned vegetables.
  - Fresh vegetables are highest in vitamins, minerals and fiber.
  - Canned vegetables have lost most of their nutritional value in the cooking and canning process.
  - Frozen vegetables can be eaten if fresh vegetables are not available.
- Vegetables can be eaten raw or cooked.
  - Some raw vegetables should be eaten every day.
  - Cooked vegetables should be lightly steamed to preserve as much of the nutrients as possible.
- Freeze the water from steaming and use later as a delicious soup stock.

Complex carbohydrates are high in fiber which
- is important for a healthy bowel
- lowers the risk of cancer, heart disease and diabetes

Fat

Fats have gotten a bad reputation in this country. As a result, a lot of "low fat" and "no fat" foods have become very popular.

It's not fat, in general that is bad for you; it's the kind of fat that you eat that you must be concerned about. A certain amount of the right kind of fat is extremely important for
- your nervous system
- your immune system
- the formation of cell membranes
- the absorption of the fat-soluble vitamins A, D, E, F, and K

Saturated fats are harmful and generally should be avoided. They contribute to elevated serum cholesterol, cancer and heart disease. Saturated fats are found in
- meat and poultry
- milk and cheese products
- chocolate products
- palm kernel oil
- coconut oil
- butter

Monounsaturated fats are healthy fats. They are found in
- most nuts
- avocados
- olive oil
- canola oil

Polyunsaturated fats contain the essential fatty acids, which are important for good health. They are found in
- sunflower seeds
- some nuts
- soybeans
- sunflower oil
- safflower oil
- fish
- flaxseed oil
- sesame oil
- wheat germ oil
- walnut oil
- corn oil

Caution: When polyunsaturated fats are highly refined and processed or partially hydrogenated, they lose their health benefits and become harmful. **Make sure all oils you use are unrefined and cold pressed or expeller pressed.**

The best oils to use are organic, cold pressed oils.
- flaxseed oil
- extra virgin olive oil
- sesame oil
- canola oil

Caution: Flaxseed oil should never be heated. Flaxseed and canola oils should always be refrigerated.

Avoid
- hydrogenated and partially hydrogenated oils
- refined oils
- vegetable shortening
- margarine
- lard

These fats contribute to
- obesity
- heart disease
- certain types of cancer

Use butter instead of margarine, but **combine the butter 50-50 with canola or sunflower oil to make better butter.** Blend it by hand or in a blender, and keep it refrigerated. Use it just like you would use butter or margarine.

Vitamins and Minerals

Vitamins are micronutrients that are
- necessary for the body's metabolic functions
- necessary for life
- generally not synthesized in the body in adequate amounts so that additional sources are usually necessary

Vitamins are either water-soluble or fat-soluble.
- Water soluble vitamins, B and C
    - are not stored in the body
    - are excreted if you take too much

- can cause deficiencies if isolated B's or ascorbic acid are taken in excess
- Fat soluble vitamins A, D, E, F and K
  - are stored in the body
  - can be harmful if you take too much

Vitamin deficiencies can cause a myriad of health problems including, but not limited to

- brittle nails
- bruising
- depression
- digestive problems
- dry hair
- dry skin
- eczema
- fatigue
- female problems
- fertility problems
- glandular malfunctions
- hair loss
- impaired immune function
- low resistance to infections
- memory loss
- muscle weakness
- nervous disorders
- poor vision
- premature aging
- sterility

Minerals occur naturally in the earth. They can be organic or inorganic. Minerals
- are essential for your body to function
- cannot be produced by your body - they must be supplied by your diet

Minerals fall into two categories:
- macrominerals
- trace minerals

The macrominerals are present in large quantities in your body, and they include
- calcium
- magnesium
- sodium
- iodine
- phosphorus
- iron
- potassium

Trace minerals are
- present in minute quantities in your body

- necessary for your body to function properly

Some of the trace minerals necessary for good health are
- boron
- copper
- selenium
- chromium
- manganese
- zinc
- cobalt
- molybdenum

Minerals
- are stored in the body
- taken in too high doses can cause toxic effects
- must be taken in the proper balance--too much of an individual mineral can cause a deficiency of another mineral

Mineral deficiencies can cause a myriad of health problems, including, but not limited to:
- anxiety
- behavioral disturbances
- constipation
- dry skin
- fatigue
- fear
- hair loss
- headaches
- hypertension
- hyperthyroid
- impaired immune function
- infertility
- insomnia
- memory loss
- menopause
- muscle spasms
- nervousness
- obesity
- premature aging
- weakness

The best way to start getting your vitamins and minerals in the proper balance is by eating plenty of fresh whole foods - fruits, vegetables, legumes and grains - every day. However, it is very difficult to get all the vitamins and minerals you need every day from the food you eat. Most of our food is grown on nutrient depleted soils and is chemically fertilized and sprayed with pesticides. **Vitamin and mineral supplements are a good way to ensure that you are getting adequate vitamins and minerals in your diet.**

Vitamin supplements can be synthetic or natural.
- Synthetic vitamins are produced in a laboratory and are chemically the same as natural vitamins, but may have harmful additives in them. Buyer beware.
- Natural vitamins may have vitamins in them that are not from food, but will not have the harmful additives that may be in synthetic vitamins.
- Vitamin supplements derived from food are going to be absorbed and utilized better than supplements not from food.

Minerals, like vitamins, can be derived from food or produced in a laboratory.
- Food based minerals are going to be better absorbed and utilized by your body.
- Minerals should not be taken with fiber supplements because fiber reduces mineral absorption in your body.

The Recommended Daily Allowance (RDA) of vitamins and minerals is the **minimum** amount necessary to prevent disease, not promote health. **To obtain and maintain optimum health, amounts of vitamins and minerals larger than the RDA are necessary.**

NUTRIENT	Adult RDA	Optimal Range
Beta Carotene		15,000-100,000 IU's
Vitamin A	5,000 IU's	10,000-25,000 IU's
Vitamin B_1	1-1.5 mg	10-500 mg
Vitamin B_2	1.2-1.6 mg	10-100 mg
Niacin	13-18 mg	50-200 mg
Niacinamide		50-500 mg
Folic Acid	400 mcg	400-800 mcg
Pantothenic Acid	4-7 mg	100 mg
Vitamin B_6	2 mg	50-100 mg
Vitamin B_{12}	3 mcg	50-500 mcg
Biotin	100-200 mcg	300 mcg
Choline		100 mg
Inositol		100 mg

PABA		25 mg
Vitamin C	45 mg	500-8,000 mg
Bioflavonoids		500 mg
Hesperidin		100 mg
Rutin		25 mg
Vitamin D	400 IU's	400 IU'S
Vitamin E	12-15 IU's	200-800 IU's
Vitamin K		70-140 mcg
Calcium	800 mg	800-1,500 mg
Magnesium	300-350 mg	400-750 mg
Potassium		99-500 mg
Iron	10-18 mg	10-30 mg
Manganese	2.5-5 mg	2-5 mg
Zinc	15 mg	30 mg
Copper	2-3 mg	2-3 mg
Chromium	80-100 mcg	200-600 mcg
Selenium	.05-.2 mg	100-400 mcg
Iodine	100-130 mcg	225 mcg
Molybdenum	.15-.5 mg	300 mcg

A good multiple vitamin/mineral supplement will help you get your vitamin and mineral intake into the optimal range. It is not advisable to do a lot of supplementing of individual vitamins or minerals without the assistance of a nutritionally oriented doctor. Many of the vitamins and minerals work together and must be in certain ratios or imbalances and deficiencies can result. Excess amounts of certain vitamins and minerals can also be toxic.

Fiber

Fiber is
- the part of the food we eat that the body cannot digest
- important for a healthy digestive tract
- found in fruits, vegetables, grains and legumes

There is no fiber in
- meat
- eggs
- dairy products

A diet low in fiber is associated with cancer and heart disease.

Water

Water is very important for a healthy body.
- Approximately 70% of your body is water.
- Water is used in just about every process that occurs in your body.
- You should drink plenty of clean, pure water to replace the water that your body uses up each day.

A **rule of thumb** to figure out how much water you should drink every day is
- one ounce of water for every 1 to 2 pounds of body weight
- take your body weight and divide it by two to get the **minimum** number of ounces of water you should drink daily

$$\frac{\text{your body weight}}{2} = \text{minimum number of ounces of water you should drink daily}$$

But you probably don't want to drink tap water because:
- No municipal water system is free of contaminants, regardless of how good the water looks, smells or tastes.
- There's no way to be sure what's in your tap water when you drink it unless you spend hundreds of dollars to have it extensively tested.
- The water coming through your tap may contain
    - pesticides, herbicides, asbestos, industrial waste
    - toxic metals such as chromium, lead, cadmium, copper
    - trace amounts of sediment, scale, dirt
    - petroleum products from oil spills
    - carcinogenic organic compounds such as benzene, ether, chloroform
- Chlorine is added to the water to kill bacteria. It reacts with organic material in the water
    - to form cancer-causing chemicals

- and may increase the risk of miscarriage to women in their first trimester of pregnancy
- In 1975, the Environmental Protection Agency (EPA) identified 253 different organic compounds in U.S. drinking water. Some of these compounds are cancer causing, some are suspected to cause cancer. Municipal water treatment systems are only required to test for a few of these chemicals.

Bottled water is not a good alternative to tap water because:
- by law, bottled water only has to be as safe as tap water
- much of the bottled water comes from the same source as your tap water
- bottlers of water have been cited for
    - not meeting water quality standards
    - keeping false records
    - adding chlorine to bottled water
- plastic from the water containers breaks down and is absorbed into the water, forming potentially toxic contaminants, and giving the water a plastic taste
- if bottled water is stored in a warm place, bacteria can grow in the water

The best way to get good, pure drinking water is to have a point-of-use filtration system in your home. That means a good quality
- water filtration system
- reverse osmosis system

Let's move on to our next stop on the road to *healthy eating.*
⇨⇨⇨

THE HEALTHY EATING FOR EXTREMELY BUSY PEOPLE FOOD PYRAMID

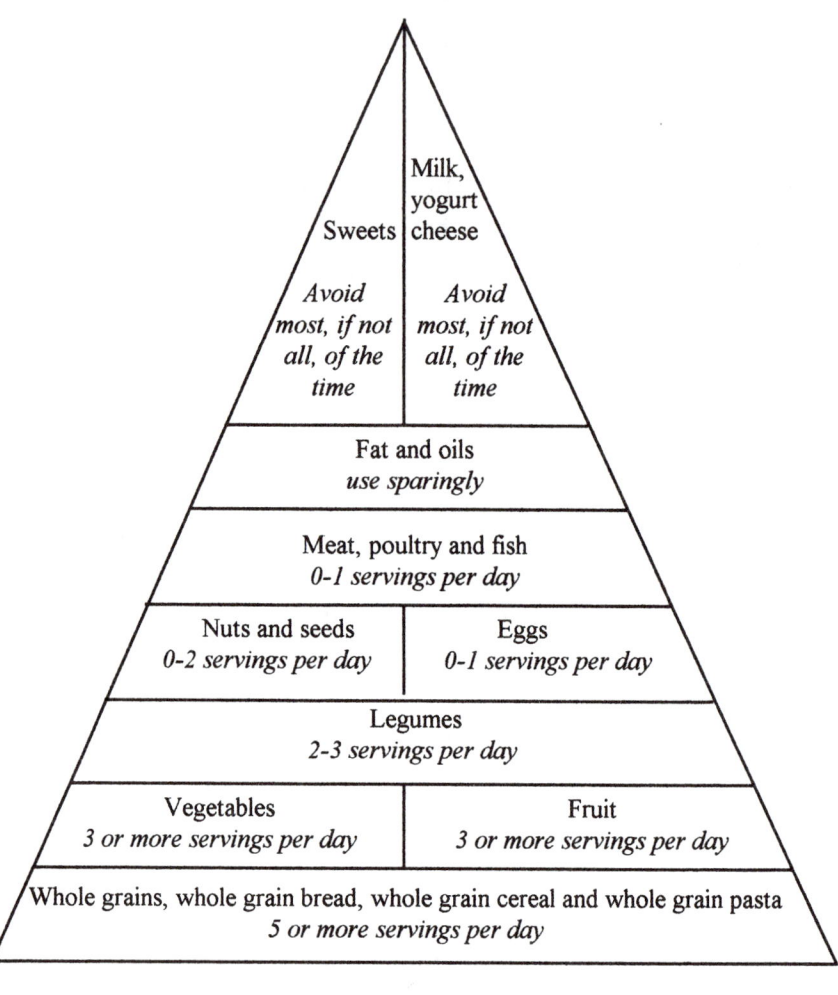

Start at the bottom and go up the pyramid. The foods you should eat the most of are at the bottom or base of the pyramid. The foods you should eat the least of are at the top.

Let's look at each group, starting at the bottom of the pyramid with whole grains, and work our way up the pyramid to the top.

Whole grains include
- amaranth
- barley
- brown rice
- buckwheat
- bulgur
- corn
- millet
- oats
- quinoa
- rye
- wheat
- wild rice

One serving of whole grains is equivalent to:
- ½ cup of cooked whole grain or hot whole grain cereal
- 1 ounce of dry whole grain cereal
- 1 slice of whole grain bread
- ½ cup of cooked whole grain pasta.

Any bread, cereal or pasta that has **enriched flour** in it, or does not say **"whole"** in front of the grain on the label is **not whole grain.**

Vegetables, organic if possible, can be fresh, frozen or canned. Choose
- fresh first
- frozen if you can't get fresh
- canned rarely or never

By eating a variety of fresh vegetables, you will be supplying your body with valuable nutrients your body needs that are not available in refined and processed foods.

One serving is equivalent to
- one cup of raw vegetables
- ½ cup of cooked vegetables.

Fruits, organic if possible, can be fresh, frozen, dried or canned. Choose
- fresh first
- frozen unsweetened with only fruit ingredients - eat frozen to avoid nutrient loss in moisture that drains off when defrosting
- sun-dried, unsweetened, unsulfured with only fruit ingredients--buy packaged, not from bulk bins that may not list added ingredients

- canned in it's own juice - eat canned rarely

One serving is equivalent to
- one medium piece of fruit,
- ½ cup of frozen fruit
- ½ cup of canned fruit
- ½ cup of cooked fruit
- ½ cup of fruit juice.

Note: 1 pound of dried fruit is made from 3-10 pounds of fresh fruit and is a concentrated source of fruit sugar, so eat sparingly.

Legumes include
- dried beans
- dried peas
- lentils
- miso
- soy milk
- chickpeas
- tempeh
- tofu

Some beans and lentils can be sprouted, and are delicious added to salads or sandwiches.

One serving is equivalent to
- ½ cup of cooked beans, peas or lentils
- 4 ounces of tofu or tempeh
- 8 ounces of soy milk.

Nuts and seeds, organic if possible
- should be eaten raw
- can be soaked to make them more digestible
    - can be blended to make nut and seed milks to substitute for dairy milk
    - can be sprouted and can be added to salads or sandwiches

If you eat whole grains, vegetables, legumes and fruits in the recommended number of servings per day, you will get sufficient protein, and

- you can eat as much as your appetite desires without ever counting calories
- you'll never have to worry about gaining weight when you eat these foods

Eggs should be from chickens that are
- fed all natural feed
- hormone and antibiotic free

One serving is 2 eggs.

If you eat **meat or poultry,**
- choose the products that come from organically grain fed, drug-free and chemical-free animals
- eat red meat not more than once a week
- remove the fat from red meat
- remove the skin from poultry

One serving is 4 ounces or less of meat or poultry

If you eat **fish**,
- choose frozen fish, it is less likely to have bacterial contamination
- eat not more than once or twice a week

One serving is 4 ounces or less.

The safest ways to cook meat or fish are
- poaching
- steaming
- roasting/baking
- stewing

Pan-frying and charcoal broiling can cause the formation of carcinogens.

Fats and oils are important to your health. **Using the right kinds of fats and oils that your body needs is as important as not using too much fat and oil.**

- Using 1-2 tablespoons of organic, unrefined flaxseed oil daily is healthy for your
    - glands
    - heart
    - immune system
    - kidneys
    - skin
- Flax oil should never be heated.
- Use flax oil on your salad with raw unfiltered apple cider vinegar and a little Celtic salt for a really tasty salad dressing.
- Use pure cold pressed sesame oil for stir-frying, it's more stable at high temperatures.
- Other good fats and oils include
    - extra virgin, first-pressed olive oil
    - cold pressed or expeller pressed sunflower oil
    - canola oil
- Combine butter 50-50 with canola oil or one of the other oils mentioned here to make "better butter."

Avoid these fats and oils and all products that contain even the smallest amount of them:
- margarine
- hydrogenated oils
- partially hydrogenated oils
- cottonseed oil
- coconut oil
- palm kernel oil
- lard

Avoid heating oils to high temperatures.

Sweets are generally made from **refined sugar**, which
- is devoid of nutrients
- uses up B vitamins and some minerals in the process of being digested, causing deficiencies

We do not need to consume any sugar at all. All the sugar that our bodies need can most efficiently be obtained from
- whole grain products
- fruits and vegetables

These foods also contain vitamins, minerals and fiber.

Milk, yogurt, cheese and all dairy products, in general, contribute to a multitude of health problems, including
- allergies
- arthritis
- asthma
- back pain
- cancer
- chronic fatigue
- common cold
- ear infections
- headaches
- heart disease
- neck pain
- obesity
- osteoporosis
- respiratory problems
- thyroid problems

Dairy products form mucous in the body which thickens, hardens and sticks to the intestinal lining, making it difficult, if not impossible for your body to absorb nutrients.

If you must use dairy products, try
- raw goat cheeses and yogurt (infrequently)
- soy yogurt

Let's shift gears now, and move on to our next stop to find out what is done to *healthy food* to make it harmful. ⇨⇨⇨

ADULTERATED FOOD: FOOD ADDITIVES, PESTICIDES AND IRRADIATION

Most of the food you find in the grocery store has been altered, adulterated or tampered with in some form to change it from it's natural wholesome state.

- Food is grown on depleted soils with chemical fertilizers and pesticides.
- It's refined and processed so that most of it's natural nutrients are removed.
- It can even be irradiated so that contaminated or spoiled food can be cleaned up and sold.

Becoming aware of these assaults to our food supply can help you avoid these undesirable foods which are dangerous to your health.

Food Additives

There are more than 3000 different chemicals purposefully added to our food supply. Testing for the safety of these chemical additives is generally done by the company that wants to produce the chemicals or to use the chemical additives in the foods they produce. The Delaney Clause of the 1958 Food Additives Amendment prohibits the addition of cancer-causing additives to food. However, because of political pressure, the FDA now allows the use of small amounts of cancer causing substances in foods.

Even if all of the additives used in our foods were safe individually, they may be harmful when combined with other additives. **Nobody knows the effects of the many different combinations of additives.**

I have listed some common food additives on the following pages. Each additive is preceded by a code representing its safety and the advisability of its use. The additive may be followed by

- some adverse effects associated with consumption of the additive
- if the additive has not been adequately tested

Here's a description of the categories used in classifying the additives.

Classification Of Food Additives

The codes below are to the left of each additive and indicate the safety of the additive.

*   GRAS - <u>G</u>enerally <u>R</u>ecognized <u>A</u>s <u>S</u>afe by the FDA.

S   There is no known toxicity. The additive appears to be safe.

A   The additive may cause allergic reactions.

C   Caution is advised. The additive may be unsafe, poorly tested, or used in foods we eat too much of.

C1 Caution is advised for certain groups in the population, such as pregnant women, infants, persons with high blood pressure, kidney problems, etc.

X   The additive is unsafe or very poorly tested.

The GRAS classification of safety by the FDA does not guarantee the additive is safe. The FDA evaluates additives based upon their ability to cause cancer and harmful reproductive effects, generally ignoring other harmful outcomes. In addition, a number of formerly GRAS additives have been removed from the GRAS list *after they were found to be harmful*. **It is virtually certain that some additives in common use now, and considered to be safe, will one day be banned.**

FOOD ADDITIVES

C   Animal or vegetable shortening - associated with heart disease, hardening of the arteries, elevated cholesterol levels.

X A Artificial color FD & C, U.S certified food color - contribute to hyperactivity in children; may contribute to learning and visual disorders, nerve damage; may be carcinogenic.

C A Artificial flavoring - may cause reproductive disorders, developmental problems; not adequately tested.

C   Aspartame - may cause brain damage in phenylketonurics; may cause central nervous system disturbances, menstrual difficulties; may affect brain development in unborn fetus.

* X A BHA - can cause liver and kidney damage, behavioral problems, infertility, weakened immune system, birth defects, cancer; should be avoided by infants, young children, pregnant women and those sensitive to aspirin.

X A Blue No. 1 - see FD&C Blue No. 1.

X A Brominated vegetable oil - linked to major organ system damage, birth defects, growth problems; considered unsafe by the FDA, can still lawfully be used unless further action is taken by the FDA.

X A BVO - see brominated vegetable oil.

* C Caffeine - psychoactive, addictive drug; may cause fertility problems, birth defects, heart disease, depression, nervousness, behavioral changes, insomnia, etc.

C   Carrageenan - may cause ulcerative colitis; suspected carcinogen.

* C1 Cream of tartar – caution if kidney or heart problems.

C   Equal - see aspartame.

X A FD&C Blue No. 1 - may cause itching, low blood pressure; may be carcinogenic; not adequately tested; see artificial color....

X A   FD&C Yellow No. 6 - causes tumors in lab animals; contaminated with carcinogens; see artificial color....

C A   Hydrogenated vegetable oil - associated with heart disease, breast and colon cancer, atherosclerosis, elevated cholesterol.

C A   Hydrolyzed vegetable protein - may cause brain and nervous system damage in infants; high salt content; may be corn, soy, or wheat based.

* C A   Modified food starch - processed with chemicals of questionable safety; not adequately tested.

* C A   Mono- & diglycerides - may be soy, corn, peanut or fat based; not adequately tested.

* C A   MSG - may cause headaches, itching, nausea, brain, nervous system, reproductive disorders, high blood pressure; pregnant, lactating mothers, infants, small children should avoid; allergic reactions common.

C A   Natural flavors - may be chemically extracted and processed and in combination with other food additives not required to be listed on the label.

X   Nitrates - form powerful cancer-causing agents in stomach; can cause death; considered dangerous by FDA but not banned because they prevent botulism.

C   Nutrasweet - see aspartame.

X   Saccharin - carcinogenic; FDA has tried to ban since 1977.

X   Sodium nitrate - see nitrates.

* C A   Sorbitol - may cause gastrointestinal distress, especially in infants and children; may be corn based.

X   Sweet'n Low - contains saccharin.

C   Vegetable broth - may contain additives not listed on the label.

For a more complete list of food additives, see **FOOD ADDITIVES: A Shopper's Guide To What's Safe & What's Not.**

Pesticides

Pesticides are chemical poisons used for destroying pests and are potentially harmful. Many pesticides are known to cause cancer. They may also cause birth defects, genetic defects or nervous system disorders.

There are two major types of pesticides:
- Contact-acting pesticides which are found on the surface of the food and may be washed or peeled off.
- Systemic pesticides which are absorbed by the plant and cannot be washed or peeled off.

There is no way for you to know what kind of pesticides are on or in the food you buy at the grocery store. You risk your health with every bite you take. The best thing you can do to reduce the amount of contact-acting pesticides you eat is to:
- thoroughly scrub all produce with a vegetable wash
- peel off the skin
- remove the outer layers of leaves

This will only remove contact-acting pesticides. **There is nothing you can do to remove systemic pesticides from the food.** In addition, peeling the skin and removing outer leaves also reduce the nutrients in the food. But even worse is that non-organic food is already much lower in nutrients than organic food.

The healthiest way to eat is to eat 100% of your food organically grown because organic foods are grown without pesticides and chemical fertilizers.

How can you tell if the food is organically grown? It will be labeled **"certified organic."** "No pesticides" does not mean organic. It may still be grown with chemical fertilizers, and be nutritionally inferior to organically grown food.

Irradiation

Irradiation is a procedure where food is exposed to low levels of radiation to
- kill pests
- make spoiled or contaminated food appear fresh
- slow ripening
- make food last longer

Irradiation destroys vitamins A, C, B1 and folic acid, and breaks down the fiber content of fruits and vegetables. It has been shown to change the taste and texture of oranges.

Animal studies on the consumption of irradiated food have documented such health problems as mutations, chromosomal damage, kidney and heart damage.

In spite of this, the FDA has approved irradiation for
- wheat and wheat flour
- potatoes
- spices
- dried vegetable seasonings
- teas
- seeds
- dried or dehydrated enzymes
- fresh pork
- fresh fruits and vegetables
- dried or dehydrated vegetable products
- poultry
- red meat

You can buy foods in the supermarket that are irradiated or have irradiated ingredients, and never know it. Irradiated food that has been processed, frozen, canned or is an ingredient in another product does not have to be listed as irradiated on the label.

Here are some food items that may have irradiated ingredients that will not be listed on the label:
- canned or frozen fruits or vegetables
- bread, may have irradiated wheat in it
- baked, canned, bottled or packaged food that has herbs or spices in it
- herbs and spices, unless the bottle says non-irradiated, they're probably irradiated

The FDA requires the radura, a symbol for irradiated food, to appear on all **fresh** foods that have been treated with irradiation. Irradiated foods are to be labeled "treated with radiation," or "treated with irradiation" and the irradiated food logo below.

How do you avoid irradiated food?
- Buy fresh organic produce.
- Buy fresh locally grown produce.
- Don't buy fresh food with the radura on it.
- Buy herbs and spices that say non-irradiated on the label.
- Buy organically grain fed, chemical free meat, poultry and eggs.

Let's move on to our next stop and find out **How To Read Labels** so you know exactly what you're eating ⇨ ⇨ ⇨

HOW TO READ LABELS

You can't rely on the packaging of a product to tell you if the product is healthy or not. Only by reading the label will you be able to tell if the food in the package is as "healthy" or as "natural" as the packaging says.

There are two pieces of information on a label that you should always read:
- Ingredients
- Nutrition information

Ingredients

It frequently appears that the manufacturer is trying to hide the ingredients in the packaged foods. They make it is difficult to find the ingredients on the label, and then be able to read them. They are often hidden under a flap of packaging material in very tiny print. **But the harder the ingredients are to find and read, usually, the more important it is that you read them.** If necessary, carry a small magnifying glass in your pocket or purse so you know exactly what is in a product before you decide to purchase it.

A general rule of thumb:
- If the list of ingredients is long, there's probably a lot of chemical additives in the product, and you're risking your health by eating it.
- If the list of ingredients is short, it may or may not have harmful additives in it, so read the ingredients carefully before you decide to purchase it.

Ingredients are listed on the label according to quantity; the ingredient making up the
- largest quantity of all the ingredients is listed first
- smallest quantity is listed last

Generally only those ingredients that are required by law to be listed on the label are listed. So, you never really know if there are any other ingredients in the product that are not listed on the label.

Watch out for statements like these on packages:
- NATURAL FRUIT FLAVORS, with Real Fruit Juice
- ALL NATURAL INGREDIENTS
- NO ARTIFICIAL PRESERVATIVES
- 100% NATURAL
- REAL FRUIT
- NO PRESERVATIVES
- NO ARTIFICIAL INGREDIENTS

Statements like these do not mean there are no harmful additives in the product. There may be harmful ingredients... The manufacturer hopes you'll think there are no harmful ingredients, but as you will see from the following examples, it's not true. Buying a product in a health food store does not guarantee that packaged products you buy will be free of harmful additives either. So, it's important to always **READ LABELS VERY CAREFULLY.**

NATURAL FRUIT FLAVORS, with Real Fruit Juice does not mean the product is only fruit juice sweetened. Here is a list of ingredients from a common breakfast cereal that would typically be eaten by kids. The front of the box says "NATURAL FRUIT FLAVORS, with Real Fruit Juice," and "Fruity Sweetened...."

Corn meal, sugar, oat flour, corn syrup, partially hydrogenated cottonseed oil, salt, grape juice concentrate, natural flavors, trisodium phosphate, yellows 5 & 6, red 40, blue 1 and other color added, vitamin C (sodium ascorbate), citric acid, a B vitamin (niacin), iron (a mineral nutrient), vitamin A (palmitate), vitamin B_6 (pyridoxine hydrochloride), vitamin B_2 (riboflavin), vitamin B_1 (thiamine mononitrate), a B vitamin (folic acid) and vitamin D.

Here is an analysis of the ingredients.

- **Sugar** is the second ingredient on the label. This means this is a very high sugar food. Sugar is "associated with blood sugar problems, depression, fatigue, B-vitamin deficiency, hyperactivity, tooth decay, periodontal disease, indigestion."
- **Corn syrup** is another form of sugar. It is the fourth ingredient on the label. This is a very high sugar food.
- **Partially hydrogenated cottonseed oil** is one of the worst oils you could consume. First of all, all partially hydrogenated oils are "associated with heart disease, breast and colon cancer, atherosclerosis, elevated cholesterol." Secondly, cottonseed oil is an irritant to the digestive tract, is high in pesticide residue and other toxic ingredients, and interferes with vitamin F functioning in the body.
- **Natural flavors** "may be chemically extracted and processed in combination with other food additives that are not required to be listed on the label."
- **Trisodium phosphate** is a cleaning product. It is an eye and skin irritant. It "can inhibit mineral absorption; may cause blood pressure, kidney disturbances, water retention."
- **Yellow No. 5** "may cause hay fever, gastrointestinal upset, skin rashes." You should avoid yellow no. 5 if you are aspirin sensitive.
- **Yellow No. 6** is unsafe. It "causes tumors in lab animals; contaminated with carcinogens."
- **Red 40** "contributes to hyperactivity in children; may contribute to learning and visual disorders, nerve damage; may be carcinogenic."
- **Blue 1** has not been adequately tested. It "may cause itching, low blood pressure; may be carcinogenic."
- **Other color added** is very vague. It doesn't say exactly what was added. Artificial colors, in general, "contribute to hyperactivity in children; may contribute to learning and visual disorders, nerve damage; may be carcinogenic."

- **Vitamin C (sodium ascorbate)** is a nutrient additive. * It is "synthetic vitamin C; may be corn based, may contribute to blood pressure, kidney disturbances, water retention."
- **Citric acid** "may erode tooth enamel; may be corn based."
- **B vitamin (niacin)** is a nutrient additive. *
- **Iron (a mineral nutrient)** is a nutrient additive. *
- **Vitamin A (palmitate)** is a nutrient additive. * It is "synthetic vitamin A; may be toxic in very large doses."
- **Vitamin B_6 (pyridoxine hydrochloride)** is a nutrient additive.*
- **Vitamin B_2 (riboflavin)** is a nutrient additive. *
- **Vitamin B_1 (thiamine mononitrate)** is a nutrient additive. *
- **B vitamin (folic acid)** is a nutrient additive. *
- **Vitamin D** is a nutrient additive. * It "may be toxic in very large doses."

* **Nutrient additives** are "nutrients added to mostly refined and processed food giving a false sense of nutritional value and can lead to nutritional imbalances; chemicals used in preparing nutrients added are not listed on the label."

So, "NATURAL FRUIT FLAVORS, with Real Fruit Juice," and "Fruity Sweetened...." **does not** mean the product is only fruit juice sweetened. In fact, grape juice concentrate is the last ingredient listed before all the chemical additives. So, it is present only in a small amount, just enough so the manufacturer can state on the label that it contains real fruit juice. In reality, it is very high in refined sugar and very low in real fruit juice. It also has more chemical ingredients than it has food ingredients. This is certainly not a food I would want to give to my child, or even eat myself.

ALL NATURAL INGREDIENTS and NO ARTIFICIAL PRESERVATIVES ADDED does not mean there are no harmful additives in the product. The ingredients from a loaf of bread that states on the label in big letters, "ALL NATURAL INGREDIENTS," and "NO ARTIFICIAL PRESERVATIVES ADDED," is listed on the next page.

Enriched wheat flour (wheat flour, malted barley, niacin, reduced iron, thiamine mononitrate, riboflavin), water, high fructose corn syrup, yeast, wheat bran, vital wheat gluten, butter. Contains 2% or less of each of the following: rye meal, corn flour, molasses, rolled whole wheat, salt, dough conditioners (ammonium sulfate, sodium stearoyl lactylate), brown sugar, honey, vinegar, oatmeal, soy flour, mono and diglycerides, partially hydrogenated soybean oil.

Here is an analysis of the ingredients.

- **Enriched wheat flour** is white flour. The bran and the germ portion of the whole wheat, which are rich in vitamins and minerals, have been refined out. To compensate for refining out approximately 20 nutrients, they add back 4 synthetic nutrients, niacin (vitamin B3), reduced iron, thiamine mononitrate (synthetic vitamin B1), and riboflavin (vitamin B2). These "nutrient additives...are added to mostly refined and processed foods giving a false sense of nutritional value and can lead to nutritional imbalances."
- **High fructose corn syrup** is basically sugar derived from corn. It is "associated with blood sugar problems, depression, fatigue, B-vitamin deficiency, hyperactivity, tooth decay, periodontal disease and indigestion."
- **Dough Conditioners**, in general, can cause mineral deficiencies.
- **Ammonium sulfate** "may cause mouth ulcers, nausea, kidney and liver problems."
- **Sodium stearoyl lactylate** may be corn, milk, peanut or soy based, and may cause blood pressure and kidney disturbances, and water retention."
- **Brown sugar** is frequently white sugar with molasses added. It is "associated with blood sugar problems, depression, fatigue, B-vitamin deficiency, hyperactivity, tooth decay, periodontal disease and indigestion."
- **Mono and diglycerides** "may be soy, corn, peanut or fat based." They may cause genetic changes, cancer, birth defects, and allergic reactions."

- **Partially hydrogenated soybean oil** is "associated with heart disease, breast and colon cancer, atherosclerosis and elevated cholesterol."

So, ALL NATURAL INGREDIENTS and NO ARTIFICIAL PRESERVATIVES ADDED **does not** mean there are no harmful additives in the product. The manufacturer hopes you'll think that, but as you can see from the above list of ingredients, it's not true.

100% Natural and Real Fruit does not mean there are no harmful additives in the product. No preservatives, no artificial ingredients does not mean there are no harmful additives in the product. Here is a list of ingredients from a frozen fruit confection that says "100% Natural" and "Real Fruit Refreshment" on the label, and "no preservatives" and "no artificial ingredients" in the list of ingredients.

Raspberries, raspberry puree, purified water, fructose, cellulose gum, guar gum, carrageenan (natural vegetable stabilizers). Made with chunks of real fruit for the health conscious lifestyle. No preservatives. No artificial ingredients.

Here is an analysis of the ingredients.

- **Fructose** is a sweetener and it's just as bad for you as sugar. In addition, it "may be corn based; may cause gastrointestinal distress, elevated cholesterol."
- **Cellulose gum** has been "shown to cause cancer in animals."
- **Guar gum** "may cause nausea, gastrointestinal upset, bloating."
- **Carrageenan** "may cause ulcerative colitis; suspected carcinogen."
  Note: The cellulose gum, guar gum, and carrageenan are listed as **natural vegetable stabilizers**. However, they are typically derived from non-edible parts of the plants, are highly processed, and contain preservatives that do not appear on the label of foods containing the gums.

- **No preservatives** are added as individual ingredients, but preservatives may be in the vegetable gums. Also, "no preservatives" does **not** mean "no chemical additives."
- **No artificial ingredients** may have been added, but that does not mean that all the ingredients are safe.

So, 100% Natural, Real Fruit Refreshment and no preservatives, no artificial ingredients **does not** mean there are no harmful additives in the product. The manufacturer even tries to convince you of that by stating "Made with chunks of real fruit for the health conscious lifestyle. No preservatives. No artificial ingredients." But as you can see from the above list of ingredients, it's not true.

Buying a product in a health food store does not guarantee that packaged products you buy will be free of harmful additives either. **The only way to be sure there are no harmful additives is to**
- buy fresh, whole organic foods
- read every label of every package you buy

FOOD ADDITIVES: A Shopper's Guide To What's Safe & What's Not is a handy little book, by this author, that you can carry around with you to help you read labels when you're shopping.

The next example is a product with no harmful ingredients.
Here is a list of ingredients from a can of Vegetarian Refried Beans from a typical grocery store.

Cooked beans, water, soybean oil, salt.

Here is an analysis of the ingredients.

All of the items on this label can be recognized as food items. There are no apparently harmful ingredients listed. This is a healthier choice than other products with a list of natural or artificial additives.

Let's just "knit pick" this apart to see if we could choose an even healthier product of this same kind.

- **Cooked beans** would be better if they were organic and the kind of beans used was named.
- **Water** is probably tap water with chlorine and other undesirable chemicals in it. Filtered water would be better.
- **Soybean oil** can be extracted with chemicals and at high temperatures. It can be refined, degummed, bleached and deodorized. Or, it can be expeller pressed at low temperatures, 85-95 degrees. Expeller pressed is best, but if it doesn't say expeller pressed on the label, it's probably not.

An ideal list of ingredients for this same product would be:

Cooked organic pinto beans, filtered water, expeller pressed organic soybean oil, sea salt (or unsalted).

Nutrition Information

Nutrition Information is more obvious on the label, but it usually doesn't give you all the information you need to interpret it.

Here's the Nutrition Information (per serving) from our cereal above with "NATURAL FRUIT FLAVORS with Real Fruit Juice."

Recommended Serving Size	1 ounce (1 cup)
Calories	110
Protein, g	1
Carbohydrates, g	25
Complex Carbohydrates, g	13
Sucrose and other sugars, g	12
Fat, g	1
Cholesterol, mg	0
Sodium, mg	140
Potassium, mg	30

PERCENTAGE OF U.S. RECOMMENDED DAILY ALLOWANCES (U.S. RDA)

Protein	2
Vitamin A	25
Vitamin C	25
Thiamine	25
Riboflavin	25
Niacin	25
Calcium	*
Iron	25
Vitamin D	10
Vitamin B6	25
Folic acid	25
Phosphorus	2
Magnesium	2
Zinc	*

* Contains less than 2% of U.S. RDA for this nutrient

It states that it provides 8 essential vitamins & iron, and is a good source of vitamin C. However,
- The 8 essential vitamins and iron added to this product are not the only vitamins and minerals your body needs.
- Adding these and ignoring the other vitamins and minerals your body needs can cause vitamin and mineral imbalances in your body and lead to deficiencies.
- Sodium ascorbate is a synthetic form of vitamin C and only a small part of the whole vitamin C complex. By consuming only a fraction of the whole vitamin C complex, you can create a vitamin C deficiency.
- "Nutrient additives," as I call the synthetic vitamins added to food products, are "nutrients added to mostly refined and processed food giving a false sense of nutritional value and can lead to nutritional imbalances; chemicals used in preparing nutrients added are not listed on the label."

What they don't tell you in the Nutrition Information, is

- 1 gram of fat = approximately 9 calories.
- 1 gram of protein = approximately 4 calories.
- 1 gram of carbohydrate = approximately 4 calories.
- 4 grams of sugar = 1 teaspoon of sugar.

To get fat calories in this example, multiply 9 calories per gram x 1 gram of fat = 9 calories from fat.

To get percentage of fat, divide 9 fat calories by 110 snack calories to get 8% fat.

Use the same procedure for protein and carbohydrate, using 4 calories per gram instead of 9.

To get the number of teaspoons of sugar in the snack, divide 12 grams of sugar in the snack by 4, to get 3 teaspoons of sugar.

The example is summarized in the chart below.

	grams	calories	percent
fat	1	9	8%
protein	1	4	4%
carbohydrate (total)	25	100	91%
sugar	12	48	44%
complex carbohydrate	13	52	47%

This cereal, **per serving**, is approximately
- 8% fat,
- 4% protein
- 91% carbohydrate
- 44% sugar, or 3 teaspoons of sugar!

Without knowing the conversion from grams to calories, and grams to teaspoons, you probably would not know that this is such a high sugar food. In addition, it is very high in sodium, and the vitamins and minerals are synthetic, and can contribute to nutrient imbalances in the body.

Here's the Nutrition Information (per serving) from a cheese-flavored snack.

Serving Size 1 ¼ ounce
Number of Servings 1

Calories	190
Protein	2 g
Carbohydrate	21 g
Fat	12 g
Cholesterol	0 mg
Sodium	390 mg
Potassium	50 mg

PERCENTAGE OF U.S. RECOMMENDED DAILY ALLOWANCES (U.S. RDA)

Protein	2
Vitamin A	*
Vitamin C	*
Thiamine	4
Riboflavin	10
Niacin	4
Calcium	*
Iron	4

* Contains less than 2% of U.S. RDA for this nutrient

Here's a summary of the nutrients:

	grams	calories	percent
Fat	12	108	58%
Protein	2	8	4%
Carbohydrate (total)	21	84	44%

This snack is approximately
- 58% fat,
- 4% protein
- 44% carbohydrate.

Without knowing the conversion from grams to calories, you probably wouldn't know this is such a high fat food. It is also very high in sodium, and very low in vitamins and minerals.

Let's take a look at how much fat is really in some "low fat" foods. If you're eating these foods because you think they're low fat, you're probably getting more fat than you bargained for.

2% Milk
- 1/2 cup of 2% milk has 50 calories and 2 grams of fat
- 2 grams of fat x 9 calories per gram = 18 fat calories
- $\frac{18 \text{ fat calories}}{50 \text{ total calories}}$ = 36% fat

Extra Lean Ground Beef
- 3 1/2 ounces of extra lean ground beef has 256 calories and is 56% fat

Skinless Chicken Breast
- 3 1/2 ounces of skinless chicken breast has 165 calories and is 22% fat.

Here's a summary in the table below.

	total calories	Grams of fat	calories from fat	percent fat
1/2 cup of 2% milk	50	2	18	36%
3 1/2 oz. extra lean ground beef	256	16	144	56%
3 1/2 oz. skinless chicken breast	165	4	36	22%

Let's move on down the road to find out how you can eat more healthfully when **Eating Out**. ⇨ ⇨ ⇨

EATING OUT

How do you know what you're eating when you eat out? You don't. But you can eat healthy food when you eat out if you choose the places where you eat carefully and ask the right questions.

- How is it cooked? Is it baked, broiled, fried, sautéed, steamed or poached? Baked, broiled, steamed and poached are the healthiest cooking methods.
- Is it cooked in a microwave? I don't recommend it.
- What's in it?
- Is it real or imitation? Real is always best.
- What spices are used? Are they irradiated? Unless you're eating at an organic, natural foods restaurant, the spices are probably irradiated.
- Do you use MSG? Ask them to "hold the MSG." If they can't, don't eat dishes that have MSG in them.
- Does it have any milk, cheese or dairy products in it?
- What kind of oil do you use? Olive oil is probably the best oil that a restaurant will use. If they don't use olive oil, it's probably a highly refined partially hydrogenated oil.
- Do you use butter or margarine? Always choose butter, never margarine.
- May I have olive oil and fresh lemon for salad dressing?
- Is it prepared fresh, or is it frozen or canned? Fresh is best, frozen next best. Avoid canned.
- Is the chicken locally grown and hormone and antibiotic free?
- Is the water tap water or filtered water? Filtered is best. Don't drink tap water.

Unless you go to a vegetarian or natural health restaurant that serves organically grown foods, you're most likely not going to get as pure quality as you're able to purchase and prepare yourself.

You're safest dishes to order are:
- Baked or steamed potatoes
- Steamed vegetables
- Garden salad with
  - olive oil and fresh lemon
  - your own salad dressing from home
  - no dressing
- Baked or broiled seafood or poultry
- Steamed rice
- Pinto or black beans cooked in water, not refried

Avoid all sauces, prepared salad dressings, soups, fried or sautéed foods, unless you're eating at a natural health restaurant where they use organically grown foods.

When you're going to be out at mealtime, you can also take your meals with you in a little ice chest. **Here's some tasty nutritious suggestions for your carry-along meals:**
- cut up vegetables
- left over salad
- sandwich on whole grain bread
- left over rice and veggies with beans or chicken chunks
- fruit snacks for 30 minutes before or 2 hours after meals

Now, let's take a side trip to **Food Combining** and see what it has to offer you. ⇨⇨⇨

FOOD COMBINING

Food combining involves eating certain kinds of foods together at a meal, and avoiding eating other kinds of foods together. Food combining is controversial. Some people swear by it saying that it enhances digestion and absorption of nutrients. Others say there is no scientific basis to support it.

Clinically, I have seen food combining work miracles in some people, and have no effect in others.

If you experience belching, flatulence, indigestion, bloating, diarrhea or constipation, you might want to consider trying to combine your foods according to the rules that follow to see if it helps you.

- ☺ Fruits should be eaten alone, 30 minutes before a meal or 2-4 hours after a meal. Melons should not be combined with any other fruit.

- ☺ Proteins combine well with non-starchy vegetables

- ☺ Starches combine well with non-starchy vegetables

- ☺ Oil combines well with starches and non-starchy vegetables

- ☹ Protein and starch do not combine

- ☹ Oil and protein do not combine

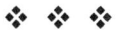

Congratulations, you've completed the first step of your *healthy eating* adventure – getting started. The next step is **taking action**—doing it consistently every day.

To assure your success, use "Your Personal Food Planner" daily. Refer to "Recommendations For Healthy Eating" frequently, especially when you make out your grocery list.

If you get discouraged because you "blew it" or you're not doing it perfectly, go back and reread "Developing Good Eating Habits That Last A Lifetime."

Every little step you take in the direction of healthier eating is going to mean a healthier you. **Keep this book handy and refer to it often.**

REFERENCES

NUTRITION ALMANAC, John D Kirschmann
NUTRITION FOR VEGETARIANS, Agatha Moody Thrash, M.D. and Calvin L. Thrash, M.D.
THE VEGETARIAN HANDBOOK, Gary Null
THE GOLDBECKS' GUIDE TO GOOD FOOD, Nikki & David Goldbeck
CLEANSE & PURIFY THYSELF, Richard Anderson, N.D., N.M.D.
PRESCRIPTION FOR DIETARY WELLNESS, Phyllis Balch, C.N.C.
DR. ATTWOOD'S LOW-FAT PRESCRIPTION FOR KIDS, Charles R. Attwood, M.D.
FOOD ADDITIVES: A Shopper's Guide To What's Safe & What's Not, Christine Hoza Farlow, D.C.
HEALTH ALERT NEWSLETTER, (vitamin C—vol. 13, issue 7, p. 6; vol. 13, issue 11, p. 8; vol. 12, issue 10, p. 6)
ROBERT CRAYHON'S NUTRITION MADE SIMPLE, Robert Crayhon, M.S.
THE WELLNESS ENCYCLOPEDIA OF FOOD AND NUTRITION, Sheldon Margen, M.D.
GET THE SUGAR OUT, Ann Louise Gittleman
MODERN NUTRITION IN HEALTH AND DISEASE, Robert Goodhart, Maurice Shils
FOOD FOR LIFE: How The New Four Food Groups Can Save Your Life, Neal Barnard, M.D.
POISONED FOOD?, Tim Lobstein, Ph.D.
FOR OUR KID'S SAKE, Anne Witte Garland
THE FOOD THAT WOULD LAST FOREVER: UNDERSTANDING THE DANGERS OF FOOD IRRADIATION, Dr. Gary Gibbs
FIT FOR LIFE, Harvey and Marilyn Diamond
NO MILK, Daniel A. Twogood, D.C.
THE BODY ECOLOGY DIET, Donna Gates
MACROBIOTIC COOKING FOR EVERYONE, Edward & Wendy Esko
AYURVEDIC COOKING FOR WESTERNERS, Amadea Morningstar
THE GARDEN OF EDEN RAW FRUIT & VEGETABLE RECIPES, Phyllis Avery
FOODS THAT CAUSE YOU TO LOSE WEIGHT: The Negative Calorie Effect, Neal Barnard, M. D.

Watch for more *KISS For Health* books coming soon.

Other books by this author:
FOOD ADDITIVES: A Shopper's Guide To What's Safe & What's Not

For information on obtaining additional copies of this or other books by this author, contact:

Dr. Christine H. Farlow
832 Lochwood Place
Escondido, CA 92026
(760) 735-8101
(760) 746-8937 fax
dfarlow@compuserve.com